THE WHOLE LIFE

HEALTH PARTNER'S GUIDE

Although the health benefits in the principles expressed in this book are well known, The Whole Life's Health Partner's Guide is neither an exercise program, diet program, nor a medical text and is not intended to replace the diagnostic expertise and medical advise of a physician. All should be certain to consult with their doctor or with a licensed health care provider before making any decisions that affect their physical health, particularly if they suffer from any medical condition or have any symptom serious enough to interfere with functioning or otherwise require treatment.

Copyright © 2019 Joshua Vazquez

All rights reserved. No portion of this book may be reproduced—mechanically, electronically, or by other means, including photocopying—without written permission of the publisher.

ISBN 978-0-578-49560-6

Written by Joshua Vazquez, Certified Health and Wellness Coach
Edited by Hope Vazquez, Certified Health and Wellness Coach
Graphic design by Robert Mason

CONTENTS

Welcome 4-5

How to be a Health Partner 7-14

Checklists 15-16

Session One: Introduction and Water 18-31

Session Two: Activity 32-39

Session Three: Nutrition 40-47

Session Four: Sleep 48-55

Session Five: Sunshine 56-63

Session Six: Fresh Air 64-71

Session Seven: Temperance 72-79

Session Eight: Trust in Divine Power 80-87

Session Nine: Hygiene 88-97

Session Ten: Maintenance 98-101

Session Eleven: Maintenance 102-105

Session Twelve: Maintenance 106-110

Notes 112-113

Work Cited 114-118

WELCOME

It brings me great joy that your eyes are gliding over the words in this book. For I know that you will be a blessing to someone in this world and plant the seeds of love in their heart. Whether you are a health professional, a pastor, or a layperson looking to minister to the needs of your family, friends, coworkers, or community, I am sure this book will give you a solid foundation to build on.

I learned to use wellness coaching as a ministry at Eden Valley Institute, where I received my certification, in 2013. Since then, I have been convinced this is the most complete approach to reach souls. This method contains every element needed to be deemed "Christ's method"— healing, teaching, preaching, relationships, and meeting felt needs.

As we follow Jesus in the Bible, we can see His method time and time again. He mingled with people and showed them He desired their good. He showed His sympathy for them and met their felt needs. He walked and talked with people, healing their diseased bodies and minds— winning their confidence. Then, He bid them, "Follow Me." This wellness coaching program facilitates every component. You will mingle with people as one who desires their good. Because of the sympathy Jesus has put in your heart, you will meet their needs. Through walking and talking you will heal body and mind and win their confidence. All the while, ever pointing them to the great Physician.

One thing I have noticed about this work is it's ability to change the culture of the local church. Each church I have worked in has come to life by the active working of the Holy Spirit. I believe God blesses this work in ways that He cannot bless many others. I believe this is the work dearest to His heart— the work of His Son.

This method has given people a better quality of life. It has strengthened relationships and built many new ones. It has caused people to quit addictions and clean up their homes. It has helped people reach heights they never thought they could. It has helped with depression and allowed happiness to take over. It has saved people from suicide and, most importantly, it has given them tangible evidence that there is a loving Savior— a Savior that is willing to heal them from the sin and suffering of this world— a God who is so loving that He sent you to help those who are crying out for The Whole Life.

I know first handed how intimidating it can be to go into a stranger's home and begin to unravel their health issues. However, it will soon become natural and you will love doing it. Especially when you seen them overcome. The wonderful part about being a Health Partner is that you don't have to teach them about the laws of health. The video and Wellness Planner will do that for you! You don't even tell them what to do. All you have to do is ask them questions and they set their goals. Your job is to listen, ask questions, encourage, and become a friend.

Does it get any easier than that?

Friend, take courage! You are embarking on a journey that will change your life as well. You will learn so much more about Jesus and His work on Earth. As you walk with people, imagine Jesus walking with those who needed His healing love. As you are encouraging those who are struggling, imagine Jesus encouraging His struggling followers. As you hear people pray for the first time, imagine Jesus hearing His disciples praying for the first time. As you live out people's testimonies with them, reminisce on the testimony Jesus has given you.

Finally, remember your success relies on your personal connection with Jesus. If you are walking with Jesus daily, and the Spirit of the living Christ is in you, people will walk with Jesus when they walk with you. Remember that holy angels are going with you and will accompany you every step of the way. Remember that Jesus will reap the harvest. Therefore, spread all the seeds of love you can and cultivate friendships that will last through eternity.

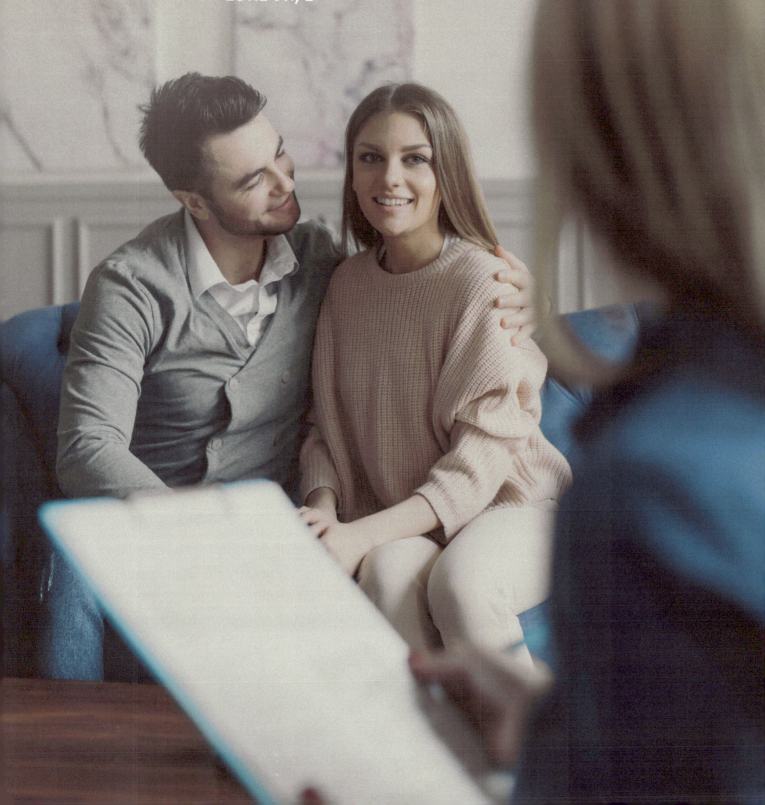

> "Then he called his twelve disciples together, and gave them power and authority over all devils, and to cure diseases. And he sent them to preach the kingdom of God, and to heal the sick."
>
> LUKE 9:1, 2

How to be a Health Partner

This Health Partner's Guide gives you step-by-step details to help you lead the twelve week Health Partnership sessions. In order to get the most benefit from this guide, there are some things we need to cover first.

This section will cover:

1. How to use this book

2. Helpful icon guide

3. How to win confidence

4. The importance of two-on-one sessions

5. Coaching two people at a time

6. The power of accountability

7. Pre-session checklist

8. Post-session checklist

How to Use This Book

This book is your Health Partner's Guide and your reference Wellness Planner. You need to bring this book with you to every session. This will help move things along as smoothly and streamlined as possible. Let's look at some of the features you'll see in this guide.

Weekly Session Guides

Each week has an individualized guide. You will need to review it completely before you arrive at your session. The guide will give you instructions for what to do before, during, and after your session. Some of the pages are only in your guide and some are what your new friend sees in their Wellness Planner.

Color Coding

In the sessions you will see colors connecting sections on opposite pages. These colors help you know where you are in this guide and where they are in their Wellness Planner.

Page Numbers

You will see two page numbers on each page. The one on the bottom right corner is the page number for this book, and the one on the bottom center is what your new friend sees in their Wellness Planner.

Open-Ended Questions

We have put sample questions you can ask in the spaces for the Wellness Vision and Weekly Goals, for you to use if you need.

ICON GUIDE

The icons below will give you instructions along the way to ensure streamlined and smooth sessions.

 This guy is your coach. He will show up when there is something important for you to do. Be sure not to pass him by.

 Whenever you see this icon, read the text provided. This will help you give clear instructions. You can use your own words to say the same thing if you feel more comfortable.

 Play the DVD.

 Pause the DVD.

 Stop the DVD.

 Go for a walk.

 Review the logs.

 It's time for them to make adjustments to their goal(s).

 It's time for them to set up a new goal(s).

Health Partner's Guide **9**

HOW TO WIN THEIR CONFIDENCE

Gaining people's confidence is crucial. There are things you can do that can make or break this process. Here are five tips to help you win their confidence.

BE ON TIME
Being on time shows people that you are dependable, have values, and that you are sensitive to their time as well.

FOLLOW THROUGH
Don't cancel unless it is an emergency or you are sick. If you cancel often, you become undependable and will lose their confidence.

LOOK PROFESSIONAL
Be sure that you and your clothes are clean and tidy. Modesty will also go a long way.

AVOID APPEARING SHOCKED
When someone shares some shocking personal information, don't look shocked or disgusted. A smile and a gentle "Okay" will reassure them that you are someone they can confide in, that you love them, and are there for them no matter what.

BE CONSISTENT
Be sure to always check all of their logs. They will appreciate your accountability and this will help them succeed.

THE IMPORTANCE OF TWO-ON-ONE SESSIONS

Here are some important reasons why you should always bring a church member or "companion" with you:

PRAYER PARTNER
Having someone praying in their mind will help you and the person being coached.

MORE CONNECTIONS
The more social connections to the church, the better. It can become a burden if you are the only one they consistently come to. Try to stick to one companion and have a couple back-up companions in case the primary companion cannot make it.

ACCOUNTABILITY
Having a companion will help make sure that no one will fall through the cracks.

SAFETY
Because we live in a sinful, immoral world, having a companion with you is extremely important for both your safety and reputation.

GOD SAID SO
See Mark 6:7 and Luke 10:1

INVOLVING YOUR COMPANION

It is important that your companion is involved in the sessions as well. Although their participation is limited, here are some ways they can be helpful:

AUDIO/VISUAL
Have your companion in charge of setting up the video and speaker and play/pause the video when needed.

READING
Include them in the reading portions of the sessions.

WALKING
When walking, try to walk with the new friend you are coaching between you both. This allows you both to connect with him/her easily.

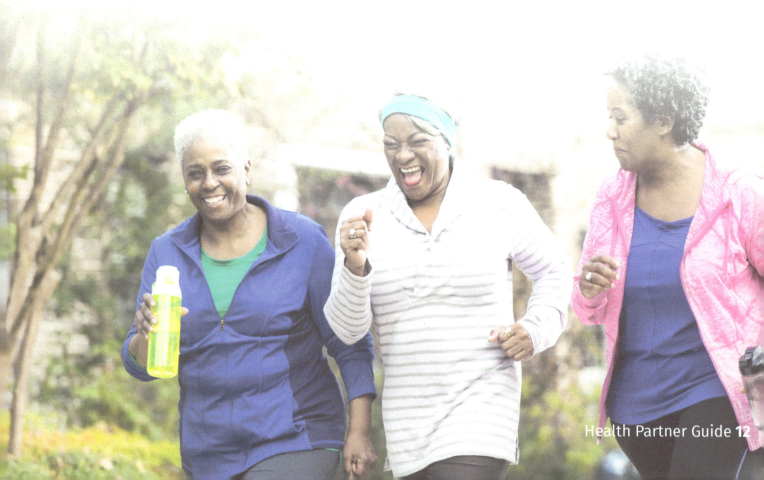

COACHING TWO PEOPLE AT A TIME

Although a two-on-one partnership is ideal, there are times when you will need to coach more than one person in a single session. Couples doing the program together is a common example. Do not coach more than two people in a single session, because the sessions become too long and impersonal.

ENCOURAGE INDIVIDUALITY
Be sure that one person is not just copying the other's goals. A gentle and good-natured, "Hey, no copying allowed. What goals can you come up with that are your very own?" could do the trick.

ONE AT A TIME
Direct your questions to one person at a time by using their names. This will maintain the "personalized" aspect of their experience.

KEEP AN ORDER
Asking the same person the questions first will help build a "rhythm" in the session. While one person is writing you can ask the other person the necessary questions.

The Power of Accountability

One of the things the person you are coaching will appreciate most is accountability. This is what the majority of people need to achieve their goals, so make sure you do not cut them short on this invaluable tool. Here are some tips to help you provide accountability for them:

Out of Sight, Out of Mind
Encourage them to place their Wellness Planner where they can see it often. Places like the refrigerator, bathroom, nightstand, or coffee table are helpful.

Check the Logs
Be sure that at each visit you check the Weekly Logs as well as Daily Meal Logs and Thankfulness logs in the back of their planner. Encourage them to fill them out if they fail to.

Go the Extra Mile
If they are struggling to meet their goals, find out why. If they are just not making them a priority, go the extra mile and help them achieve them. For example, if they are not getting active during the week, offer to go with them as often as you can. This will help them be accountable and will encourage them to do it.

PRE-SESSION CHECKLIST

Use this checklist before each section to make sure you have what you need. The "Bring This" items are what you need to bring each session. If there is a particular session that requires you to bring something special, we will let you know in that week's session checklist.

BRING THIS

- [ ] Your Health Partner's Guide
- [ ] 2 Wellness Planners
- [ ] "8 Laws" DVD
- [ ] Extra pens and pencils
- [ ] Portable DVD player/Laptop and speaker

BE PREPARED

- [ ] Review any information you have on your new friend.
- [ ] Review each session completely.
- [ ] Pray before you leave to go to the appointment.
- [ ] Check all electronics to make sure they are charged and working.
- [ ] Have the "8 Laws" DVD loaded and ready to play the segment for that session.

POST-SESSION CHECKLIST

Once you leave your session, there are some things you should do to help you succeed. Here are some important pointers:

JOT IT DOWN
Write down important information that you learned about your new friend in the session: Names of family members, pets, hobbies, prayer requests, etc. Also, important dates like their anniversary, birthday, doctor's appointments, etc. Knowing these and asking them about their kids, appointments, or congratulating them on their anniversary will help you build a good relationship.

PRAY
It is key that you envelop your session in prayer.

GET THE ANSWER
Did your new friend ask you a question you didn't know the answer to? That is OK! Just make sure you do your best to find the answer before your next session. Check several sources to make sure what you tell them is 100 percent accurate.

"The Lord bless thee, and keep thee: The Lord make his face shine upon thee, and be gracious unto thee: The Lord lift up his countenance upon thee, and give thee peace. And they shall put my name upon the children of Israel; and I will bless them." — I AM

SESSION ONE
WATER

Target time: 1.5 – 2.0 Hours

The Whole Life Health Partner's Guide

BE PREPARED

- ☐ Review the Pre-Session Checklist on page 15 of this guide.
- ☐ Review any information you have on your new friend.
- ☐ Review Session One completely.
- ☐ Check all electronics to make sure they are charged and working.
- ☐ Pray before you leave to go to the appointment.
- ☐ Videos to play: Introduction & Water
- ☐ Bring a BPA free water bottle.

Upon Arrival

Make sure you and your companion know their name before you come to the door. Come to the door with a smile. Once they open the door, introduce yourself again. Give them a warm greeting and ask them how they are doing.

Be pet-friendly. If they have a friendly dog or a sweet kitty, be sure to be friendly with them as well. This will often help with the awkwardness that comes with being in a stranger's home and, for them, having a stranger in their home.

INTRODUCTION AND INSTRUCTIONS

 DO THIS:

1. Get to know them a little. Find out how long they have lived in the area and where they lived before. Do they have any children or grandchildren? What do they do for work? If they are retired, what was their career? If you have any connections with their answers, build on them.

2. Tell them how excited you are that they are going to experience The Whole Life that you are experiencing or on the journey to experiencing. Say this:

 "I am excited that you are starting your journey to experience The Whole Life. I want to remind you that this is a minimum twelve session program. This means that you will meet with us for twelve sessions over a twelve-week period. However, if you miss a week, the program is now thirteen weeks long. This allows you to take advantage of all twelve sessions. This is only the minimum, and I want you to know that I am here for you as long as you need me — with no obligation. It is always just the cost of the Wellness Planner. This session is going to be the longest session because we have a lot to figure out. It will be about one and a half to two hours. The following sessions will be thirty minutes to an hour."

3. Give them their Wellness Planner and say this:

 "This is your Wellness Planner. It is $30. This is where you will write your goals, struggles, and solutions. This is also where you will log all of your progress and keep track of your wellness journey. The first nine sessions will touch on different health principles and the last three sessions are to help you maintain your momentum.

If you have any questions, feel free to ask. Let's get you started by turning to page 5. I will read the first paragraph and we can alternate reading, is that okay with you?"

Your Journey to The Whole Life Begins Today

HOW THE PROGRAM WORKS

Have you ever started a diet or workout only to stop after a few days? We know the struggle. This program is unique because instead of focusing on achieving results as soon as possible, we help you achieve your own wellness goals in small, attainable steps that will ensure life-long results. It is meant to be tailored to your specific needs, and help you achieve health and wholeness in every aspect of your life. No crash diets or demanding workouts required here. Are you ready for the Whole Life? Your journey begins today!

Two Page Numbers?
The one on the bottom right hand corner refers to this guide and the one in the center of the page refers to their Wellness Planner.

YOUR WELLNESS VISION

Imagine a staircase. At the top are ten health goals you want to accomplish. These ten health goals are what make up your personal "Wellness Vision"—your perfect picture of health. Once you achieve those ten goals, you have reached your Wellness Vision, the top of the staircase. Some people have small staircases and some larger staircases. The size of yours will indicate how long your journey will be.

WEEKLY GOALS

The weekly goals are like single steps on the staircase. They are small, yet they get you where you need to go. Your rate of progress depends on how well you accomplish your weekly goals. They are the make-or-break factor in this staircase. Accomplish your weekly goals, and you are guaranteed to get top-notch results!

SETTING GOALS

Your goals need to be **SMART**. SMART is an acronym for **S**pecific, **M**easurable, **A**ttainable, **R**elative, and **T**ime-Sensitive.

EXAMPLES OF WEEKLY GOALS
I will do a cardio workout for 10 minutes, 3 days per week.
I will eat 3-4 servings fruits and veggies, 3 days per week.

Another important factor to remember when setting goals is your choice of words. Avoid "I will try…", "I would like to…", "…when I can", etc. Words are powerful and impact the action you take toward your goals. You should always start your goals with "I will…". Let's get started!

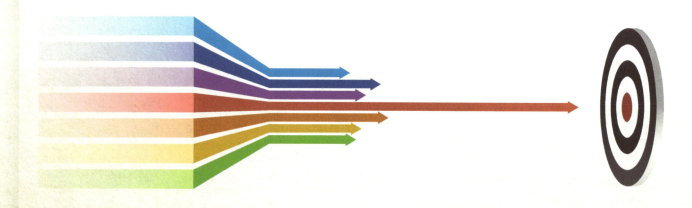

"Do you have any questions before we move on?"

 If they have questions, answer them. Then say this:

"Now we are going to watch a short video about eight of the nine laws of health. If you use these principles, you will reach your optimal potential for health and wellness."

 **Push play on your laptop or DVD player.
Only play the Introduction video.**

 Pause the video.

READ ME: "Let's begin by filling out the following sections, on page 8, one at a time. We will begin by casting your Wellness Vision.

"Your Wellness Vision is who you ultimately want to be and what you want to be doing when you reach the top of your staircase. Once you reach these goals, all you will have to do is maintain the habits that have become your lifestyle!" *

*Italics indicate direct quotes from the Wellness Planner on the corresponding page.

SAMPLE QUESTIONS

What does ideal wellness look like for you personally?

What are some things that you would like to be doing regularly that are difficult for you to do now?

How would you like to see yourself at the end of the 12 session program?

Remember, silence after asking questions is golden. Let them do the thinking and the talking once you've asked your question. Also, make sure their goals are **S.M.A.R.T.** Once they are done figuring out their vision, move on to the **My Obstacles** section.

READ ME: "Now, let's discover your obstacles. *What events, circumstances, or habits are standing in the way of reaching your Wellness Vision?*"

Once they are done figuring out their obstacles, move on to the **My Strategies to Overcome My Obstacles** section.

READ ME: "Now, that we know what your obstacles are, we can figure out some strategies to overcome them. *What are some new methods or habits that will help you overcome your obstacles?*"

Once they are done figuring out their strategies, move on to the **My Motivators** section.

Health Partner's Guide 24

WELLNESS VISION

Your Wellness Vision is who you ultimately want to be and what you want to be doing when you reach the top of your staircase. Once you reach these goals, all you will have to do is maintain the habits that have become your lifestyle!

MY WELLNESS VISION IS

OBSTACLES

What events, circumstances, or habits are standing in the way of reaching your Wellness Vision?

MY OBSTACLES ARE

STRATEGIES

What are some new methods or habits that will help you overcome your obstacles?

MY STRATEGIES TO OVERCOME MY OBSTACLES ARE

READ ME: "Let's move on to the My Motivators section. *What will motivate you to stay on track? Is it longevity with your family and friends, losing a few pant sizes, fighting disease, or something else?*"

Once they are done figuring out their motivators, move on to the My Support System section.

READ ME: "Finally, let's move to the My Support System section. *Are there any people, organizations, or clubs that you are affiliated with that will support you in your wellness journey?*"

NEXT:

Push play on your laptop or DVD player. Only play the **Water** video.

Stop the video when it finishes. There are no more videos in this session. **Give them the bottle of water**.

Health Partner's Guide **26**

MOTIVATORS

What will motivate you to stay on track? Is it longevity with your family and friends, losing a few pant sizes, fighting disease, or something else?

MY MOTIVATORS ARE

_____

_____

_____

SUPPORT SYSTEM

Are there any people, organizations, or clubs that you are affiliated with that will support you in your wellness journey?

MY SUPPORT SYSTEM

People: _____

Organizations/Clubs: _____

SESSION ONE
WATER

- Review the key points from the video. You should take turns reading them.

- Have them fill out these two sections.

- Have them read the **Three Tips for Success**.

> "Basically **not drinking enough water** can be as harmful to your heart as **smoking**..." [1]
> — Dr. Jacqueline Chan

Health Partner's Guide 28

Water, if taken in recommended amounts, will cure or significantly reduce kidney stones, gallbladder disease, constipation, urinary track infections, high blood pressure, glaucoma, and venous blood clots. [2], [3], [4], [5], [6], [7], [8]

How are your current water drinking habits affecting your health?

_____

_____

_____

How will drinking more water affect your current health?

_____

_____

_____

Three tips to help you succeed in week one:

1. Keep this planner in a place you frequent, such as the kitchen, the bathroom, or on your nightstand.

2. Track your progress by logging on page 31.

3. Drink your water when you wake up, 15 minutes before meals, 1–1 ½ hours after meals, and before bedtime. This will help you create a hydrating schedule.

The water formula: $\frac{\text{Weight}}{2}$ = Ounces

Your body is 75% water.

Your brain is 85% water

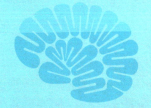

"**Brain cells** need two times more energy than other cells in the body. **Water** provides this energy more effectively than **any other** substance."
— Dr. Corinne Allen

11

Health Partner's Guide 29

Have them turn to page 31 and set up their water goal for that week. Find out how much water they are drinking now and how much they would like to add to that amount. Make sure their goal is **S.M.A.R.T.**

 SUGGESTED QUESTIONS FOR GOAL SETTING:

How much water do you currently drink every day?

How much water would you like to add to what you are currently drinking?

What do you need to do to make this happen?

 Point to them on page 31 where they will log the amount of water they drink each day. **Tip:** Suggest that they can use a specific water bottle or cup to keep track of their ounces. If they don't know how many ounces the cup or bottle is, they can fill it up and pour it into a measuring cup to figure out the ounces.

 WRAP IT UP! The session is almost over.

 READ ME: "That is all for today. I am so excited that you are on your way to experience The Whole Life. All you need to work on this week is drinking water. **Next week, We are going to start walking together, so be sure to wear some shoes that you are comfortable walking in.**"

 Confirm the day and time for next week. Give a warm, friendly goodbye. The session is now over.

 Once you leave, complete the Post-Session Checklist on page 16 of this guide.

Week One

What is your water goal for this week?

_____

_____

Daily Water Log

Example of Daily Water Log

65 oz.	65 oz.	65 oz.	70 oz.	70 oz.	75 oz.	75 oz.

Ask the Coach

_____

_____

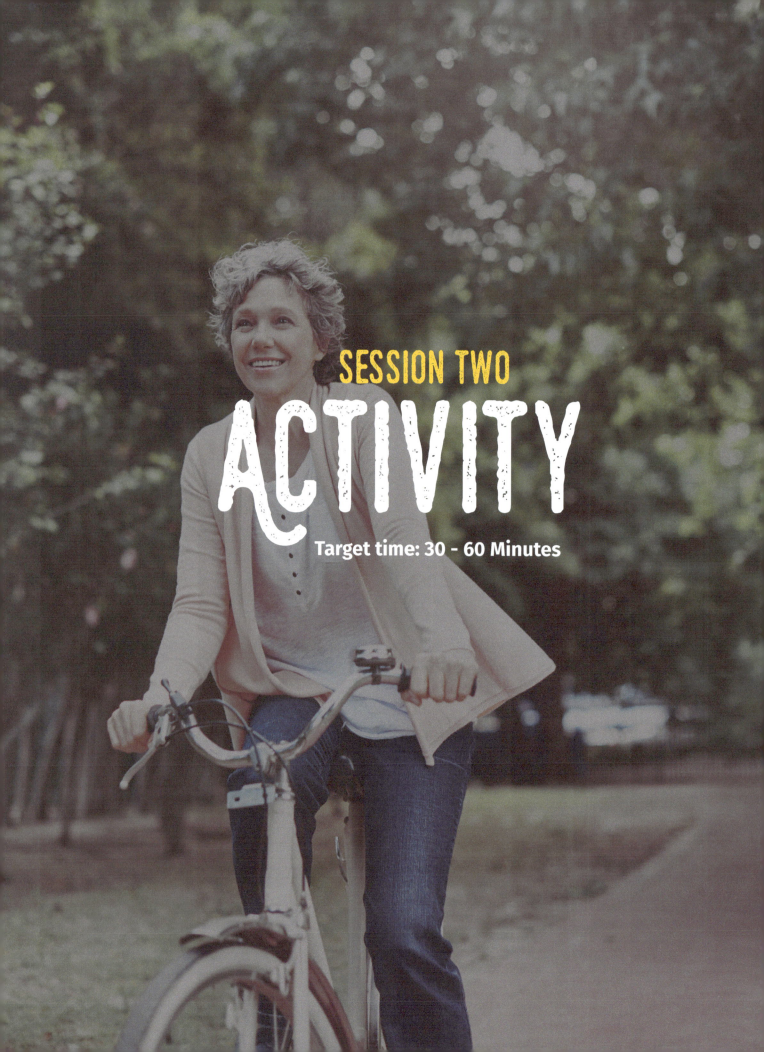

The Whole Life Health Partner's Guide

 ## BE PREPARED

- ☐ Review the Pre-Session Checklist on page 15 of this guide.

- ☐ Review any information you have on your new friend.

- ☐ Review Session Two completely.

- ☐ Check all electronics to make sure they are charged and working.

- ☐ Pray before you leave to go to the appointment.

- ☐ Video to play: Exercise

- ☐ **Bring your walking shoes.**

Upon Arrival

Make sure you and your companion know their name before you come to the door. Come to the door with a smile. Once they open the door, introduce yourself again. Give them a warm greeting and ask them how they are doing.

Set your things at the table and let them know you are going for a walk first thing. **Say this:**

SAY THIS: "We are going to walk first thing today. **We will walk at your pace, so whenever you feel like you need to turn around and come back, we will turn around and come back.** We are going to use this walk to gauge your activity goal for this week."

It's time for a walk. Pay attention to how far they walk and use this to guide their activity goal for this week. For example, if they struggle with one lap around the block, a goal of five or ten may be far-fetched.

This is a wonderful time to get to know them on a personal level and build a friendship. Be open with them and they will be open with you. At this point, do not bring up your faith unless they ask you a question that leaves you no other choice.

Log Review

Once you are back from your mind-stimulating walk, review their water log from the previous week on **page 31**. Congratulate them if they met their goals.

IF THEY DID NOT MAKE THEIR GOAL(S), SAY THIS:

"I'm sorry you didn't complete your goal. Don't be discouraged though. Making changes can be difficult at first, but you will get there. This program is tailored to go at your pace. Do you think your goal was too big?"

If yes, ask them if they would like to change the goal to something they know they can do this week.

If no, ask them if they want to keep the same goal and try it again this week.

Set the water goal for this week on page 32.

Push play on your laptop or DVD player. Only play the Exercise video.

Stop the video when it finishes.
There are no more videos in this session.

Health Partner's Guide **35**

- Review the key points from the video. You should take turns reading them.

- Have them fill out these two sections.

- Have them read the **Four Tips for Success**.

60 For every minute of exercise, you gain two minutes of longevity.[1]

Health Partner's Guide **36**

Physical fitness is the most important predictor for longevity.[2]

Regular physical activity decreases the risk for many diseases including obesity, high blood pressure, coronary heart disease, stroke, diabetes, osteoporosis, many cancers, anxiety, and depression.[3]

Staying fit increases your lifespan more than quitting smoking![4]

HOW ARE YOUR CURRENT ACTIVITY HABITS AFFECTING YOUR HEALTH?

HOW WILL BEING MORE PHYSICALLY ACTIVE AFFECT YOUR CURRENT HEALTH?

FOUR TIPS TO HELP YOU SUCCEED IN WEEK TWO:

1. Use tips 1-3 from week one.

2. Break up your activity into multiple segments throughout the day. For example, if your goal is to walk 30 minutes each day, you could walk 10 minutes morning, noon, and evening.

3. Decide where you would enjoy doing your activity the most. Do you prefer to count laps at a track, or do you like to walk in the woods or on the beach? Going to a place you enjoy will encourage you to stick to your goal.

4. Have a back-up plan. If your routine activity is outside, what will you do if there is bad weather?

5.7 YEARS

People who remain physically active remain disability-free for an additional 5.7 years.[5]

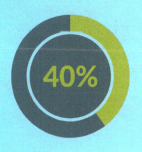

40%

The most physically active breast cancer patients reduce the risk of cancer-related deaths and recurrence by up to 40%.[6]

Health Partner's Guide 37

Have them use today's walk as their gauge for this week's activity goal. **They will set their goal on page 32** of the Wellness Planner. Make sure their goal is **S.M.A.R.T.**

 SUGGESTED QUESTIONS FOR SETTING GOALS:

How often are you active?

How many times this week will you walk the distance we walked today?

What do you need to do to make this happen?

What is your backup plan?

 Show them on page 32 where they will log this week's progress.

 WRAP IT UP! The session is almost over.

 READ ME: "That is all for today. All you need to work on this week is drinking water and being active. **We are going to continue walking together each week."**

 Confirm the day and time for next week. Give a warm, friendly goodbye. The session is now over.

 Once you leave, complete the Post-Session Checklist on page 16 of this guide.

Health Partner's Guide 38

Week Two

What is your water goal for this week?

Daily Water Log

What is your activity goal for this week?

Daily Activity Log

Example of Daily Activity Log

.5 mi.	.5 mi.	.75 mi.	20 min.	20 min.	25 min.	30 min.

Ask the Coach

Health Partner's Guide

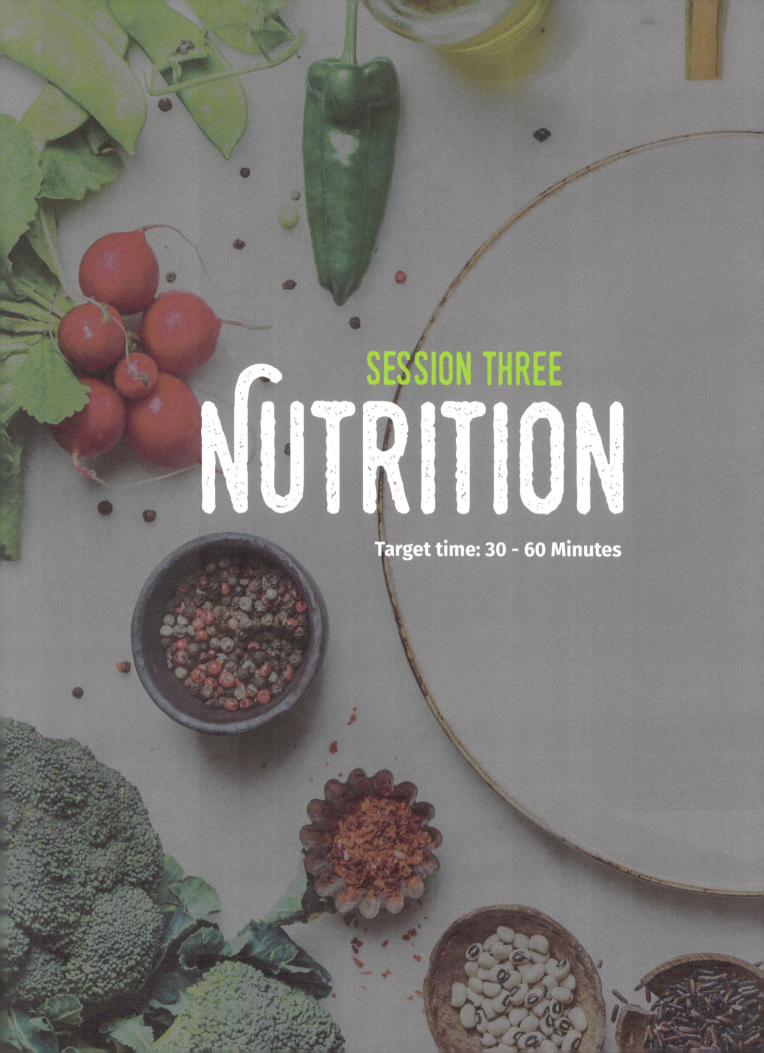

SESSION THREE
NUTRITION
Target time: 30 - 60 Minutes

The Whole Life Health Partner's Guide

BE PREPARED

- ☐ Review the Pre-Session Checklist on page 15 of this guide.

- ☐ Review any information you have on your new friend.

- ☐ Review Session Three completely.

- ☐ Check all electronics to make sure they are charged and working.

- ☐ Pray before you leave to go to the appointment.

- ☐ Video to play: Nutrition

- ☐ **Bring your walking shoes.**

UPON ARRIVAL

Make sure you and your companion know their name before you come to the door. Come to the door with a smile. Once they open the door, give them a warm greeting and ask them how they are doing.

It's time for a walk. Don't forget, this is a wonderful time to get to know them on a personal level and build a friendship. Be open with them and they will be open with you. At this point, they might ask you about your faith. Just because they ask, it doesn't mean it's the right time to go into detail. Perhaps a simple "I'm a Christian" is appropriate. Let the Lord lead you.

Log Review

Once you are back from your mind-stimulating walk, review their water log from the previous week on **page 32**. Congratulate them if they met their goals.

IF THEY DID NOT MAKE THEIR GOALS, SAY THIS:

"I'm sorry you didn't complete your goal. Don't be discouraged though. Making changes can be difficult at first, but you will get there. This program is tailored to go at your pace. Do you think your goal was too big?"

If yes, ask them if they would like to change the goal to something they know they can do this week.

If no, ask them if they want to keep the same goal and try it again this week.

Set the water and activity goal for this week on page 33.

Push play on your laptop or DVD player. Only play the Nutrition video.

Stop the video when it finishes.
There are no more videos in this session.

- Review the **11 Great Habits to Learn** from the video. You should take turns reading them.

- Have them fill out these two sections.

- Have them read the **Five Tips for Success.**

NUTRITION

Food is the fuel your body needs to run properly. Just like your vehicle, your body's performance relies on what you put into your tank. You wouldn't want to put low performance fuel into a Lamborghini or gasoline into a diesel. The results could be disastrous.

HOW ARE YOUR CURRENT EATING HABITS AFFECTING YOUR HEALTH

HOW WILL EATING MORE NUTRITIOUS FOODS AFFECT YOUR CURRENT HEALTH?

SIX TIPS TO HELP YOU SUCCEED IN WEEK THREE:

1. Don't concentrate on what you need to take away from your diet. Think about all of the wonderful foods you get to add to your diet.
2. Learn to read food labels.
3. Make a list of your favorite healthy foods and add them to your shopping list.
4. Find some healthy, tasty recipes.
5. Make a meal plan for the week.
6. Complete the daily meal logs beginning on page 59.

Here are 11 great habits to learn:[1]

1. Learn to read food labels.
2. Eat a large breakfast.
3. Eat 75% your calories in the first two meals, breakfast and lunch.
4. Have only a light meal in the evening, such as soup, cereal, or a small sandwich—mainly foods that are easy to digest.
5. Remember to drink plenty of water.
6. Consume 10 servings of fruits and vegetables each day.
7. Eat a level handful of nuts each day.
8. Eliminate snacks. 20% of all calories now come from snack foods in America.
9. Choose whole grains such as whole wheat bread, whole-grain cereals, and red, black, or brown rice.
10. Avoid sugar-sweetened beverages including fruit juice.
11. Eat more legumes.

Calories	Sodium	Salt	Sugar
300	225	0.5g	25g
12%	12%	2%	5%

Health Partner's Guide **45**

Have them set this week's nutrition goal on page 33 of the Wellness Planner. They can use the 11 great habits on page 15 if they want. Make sure their goal is **S.M.A.R.T.**

 SUGGESTED QUESTIONS FOR SETTING GOALS:

What positive changes will you make this week to your current diet?

What are some healthy foods you would like to add to your meals?

What do you need to do to make this happen?

 Show them the meal log on page 59. Let them know they need to fill this out as detailed as possible. **This is a great time to ask them if they want to cook some recipes together.**

 WRAP IT UP! The session is almost over.

 READ ME: "That is all for today.. **We are going to continue walking together each week."**

 Confirm the day and time for next week. Give a warm, friendly goodbye. The session is now over.

 Once you leave, complete the Post-Session Checklist on page 16 of this guide.

Week Three

What is your water goal for this week?

Daily Water Log

What is your activity goal for this week?

Daily Activity Log

What is your Nutrition goal for this week?

Daily Nutrition Log (Also use the daily meal log on page 59.)

Example of Daily Nutrition Log (Corresponds with the 11 great habits on page 15.)

1, 2, 5, 10	1, 2, 5, 10	2, 3, 5, 10	2, 3, 5, 10	2, 3, 4, 5, 10	2, 3, 4, 5, 10, 11	2, 3, 4, 5, 10, 11

Ask the Coach

Health Partner's Guide

SESSION FOUR
SLEEP
Target time: 30 - 60 Minutes

The Whole Life Health Partner's Guide

 ## BE PREPARED

- ☐ Review the Pre-Session Checklist on page 15 of this guide.
- ☐ Review any information you have on your new friend.
- ☐ Review Session Four completely.
- ☐ Check all electronics to make sure they are charged and working.
- ☐ Pray before you leave to go to the appointment.
- ☐ Video to play: Rest
- ☐ **Bring your walking shoes.**

Upon Arrival

Come to the door with a smile. Give them a warm greeting and ask them how they are doing.

 It's time for a walk. Don't forget, this is a wonderful time to get to know them on a personal level and build a friendship. Be open with them and they will be open with you. At this point, they might ask you about your faith. Let the Lord lead you.

 Log Review

Once you are back from your walk, review their weekly logs from the previous week on **page 33. Don't forget to check their meal log**. Congratulate them if they met their goal(s).

 IF THEY DID NOT MAKE THEIR GOAL(S) SAY THIS:

"I'm sorry you didn't complete your goal(s). Don't be discouraged though, making changes can be difficult at first but you will get there. Do you think your goal(s) was too big?"

 If yes, ask them if they would like to change the goal(s) to something they know they can do this week.

 If no, ask them if they want to keep the same goal(s) and try it again this week.

 Set the water, activity, and nutrition goals for that week on page 34.

 Push play on your laptop or DVD player. Only play the **Sleep** video.

 Stop the video.
There are no more videos in this session.

Health Partner's Guide 51

SESSION FOUR
SLEEP

- Review the key points from the video. You should take turns reading them.

- Have them fill out these two sections.

- Have them read the **Seven Tips for Success.**

People with little sleep tend to be more overweight and have shorter lifespans.[1], [2]

Health Partner's Guide 52

Newborns need 16-18 hours of sleep, young children 10-12 hours, older children and teens 9 hours, adults 7-8 hours, and seniors 9 hours.[3]

Good sleepers are mentally sharper and also at lower risk of neurological diseases such as Alzheimer's.[4], [5]

LESS THAN 7

If you sleep less than seven hours each night, your immune system would suffer for it. This makes you three times more likely to get sick.[6]

HOW ARE YOUR CURRENT SLEEPING HABITS AFFECTING YOUR HEALTH?

_____

_____

_____

HOW WILL SLEEPING THE APPROPRIATE AMOUNT OF HOURS AFFECT YOUR CURRENT HEALTH?

_____

_____

_____

_____

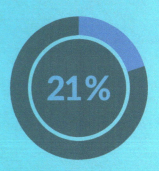

It has been shown that for adults sleeping less than seven hours, their risk of dying increases by 21% in women and 26% in men.[7]

SEVEN TIPS TO HELP YOU SUCCEED IN WEEK FOUR:

1. Turn off lights and noise. Exposure to light after dusk reduces melatonin levels by 71%. Avoid all electronic screens just before bedtime.[8]
2. Stick to a schedule that gets you to bed well before midnight.
3. Relax and get comfortable.
4. Say no to sleeping pills. They inhibit your body's ability to achieve optimal REM sleep.[9]
5. Eat a light meal at least 2-3 hours before bedtime.
6. Accomplish your daily activity goal hours before bedtime.
7. Write down 5 things you are thankful for each night and don't go to bed angry.

Health Partner's Guide 53

Have them set this week's sleep goal on **page 35** of the Wellness Planner. They can use the 7 tips in their planner on page 17 if they want. Make sure their goal is **S.M.A.R.T.**

 SUGGESTED QUESTIONS FOR SETTING GOALS:

How much sleep do you get now?

How much sleep can you add to your nightly routine?

What do you need to do to make this happen?

 Show them the thankfulness log on page 69. Let them know they can write down anything they are thankful for, no matter how big or small.

At the end of the week they can list the top five things they are thankful for on page 35.

 WRAP IT UP! The session is almost over.

 READ ME: "That is all for today. I want to remind you to complete the all of the logs this week. It is very important for us to see and track all of your progress."

 Confirm the day and time for next week. Give a warm, friendly goodbye. The session is now over.

 Once you leave, complete the Post-Session Checklist on page 16 of this guide.

Health Partner's Guide 54

What is your sleep goal for this week?

_____

_____

Daily Sleep Log

The top five things I am thankful for this week (from thankfulness log on page 69):

_____

_____

_____

Example of Daily Sleep and Thanksgiving Log

6.5 hrs.	6.5 hrs.	7 hrs.	7 hrs.	7.5 hrs.	7.5 hrs.	8 hrs.
I am thankful for: Making my water goal, the sunshine today, the new recipe we had for breakfast, good sleep I had last night, and my family.							

ASK THE COACH _____

_____

Health Partner's Guide

SESSION FIVE
SUNLIGHT

Target time: 30 - 60 Minutes

The Whole Life Health Partner's Guide

BE PREPARED

- ☐ Review the Pre-Session Checklist on page 15 of this guide.
- ☐ Review any information you have on your new friend.
- ☐ Review Session Five completely.
- ☐ Check all electronics to make sure they are charged and working.
- ☐ Pray before you leave to go to the appointment.
- ☐ Video to play: Sunlight
- ☐ **Bring your walking shoes.**

Upon Arrival

Come to the door with a smile. Give them a warm greeting and ask them how they are doing.

 It's time for a walk. Don't forget, this is a wonderful time to get to know them on a personal level and build a friendship. Be open with them and they will be open with you. At this point, they might ask you about your faith. Let the Lord lead you.

 Log Review

Once you are back from your walk, review their weekly logs from the previous week on **pages 34 and 35. Don't forget to review their meal log. Have them show you that they completed the thankfulness log. This may be private so just check for completion.** Congratulate them if they met their goal(s).

 IF THEY DID NOT MAKE THEIR GOAL(S) SAY THIS:

"I'm sorry you didn't complete your goal(s). Don't be discouraged. You are making progress, and you will get there. Do you think your goal(s) was too big?"

 If yes, ask them if they would like to change the goal(s) to something they know they can do this week.

 If no, ask them if they want to keep the same goal(s) and try it again this week.

 Set the water, activity, nutrition, and sleep goal for that week on pages 36 and 37.

 Push play on your laptop or DVD player. Only play the **Sunlight** video.

 Stop the video.
There are no more videos in this session.

Health Partner's Guide

Health Partner's Guide 59

Review the key points from the video. You should take turns reading them.

 Have them fill out these two sections.

 Have them read the **Three Tips for Success.**

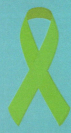 *Sunshine is important for cancer reduction, rickets prevention, and reducing osteoporosis.*[1], [2], [3]

Phototherapy changes the chemistry of the brain while boosting Vitamin D levels.[4]

Seasonal Affective Disorder or SAD is caused by decreasing amounts of sunshine and colder weather.[5]

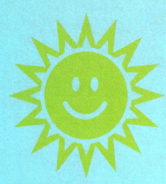

How is the amount of sunshine you are getting now affecting your health?

How will getting 20-30 minutes of sunshine each day affect your current health?

Sunshine can help keep you happy and fight depression![4]

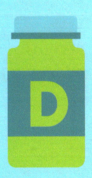

THREE TIPS TO HELP YOU SUCCEED IN WEEK FIVE:

1. Exercise outside. If you are exercising for 20-30 minutes outdoors in the sunshine, you will meet your goal.
2. Don't get sunburned. This will definitely keep you from meeting your daily goal.
3. Purchase a light box if you live in a place where the sun doesn't shine often.

Vitamin D can help turn on good genes while suppressing bad genes, especially cancer-promoting genes.[4]

Health Partner's Guide **61**

Have them set this week's sunlight goal on page 37 of the Wellness Planner. Make sure their goal is **S.M.A.R.T.**

SUGGESTED QUESTIONS FOR SETTING GOALS:

How much sunlight do you get now?

How much sunlight can you add to your daily routine?

How will you add sunlight for that amount of time?

WRAP IT UP! The session is almost over.

READ ME: "That is all for today. Be sure and complete all of the logs this week. It is very important for us to see and track all of your progress."

Confirm the day and time for next week. Give a warm, friendly goodbye. The session is now over.

Once you leave, complete the Post-Session Checklist on page 16 of this guide.

Health Partner's Guide

What is your sleep goal for this week?

_____

_____

Daily Sleep Log

The top five things I am thankful for this week (from thankfulness log on page 70):

_____

_____

_____

What is your sunshine goal for this week?

_____

_____

Daily Sunshine Log

Example of Daily Sunshine Log

10 min.	10 min.	15 min.	15 min.	20 min.	25 min.	30 min.

ASK THE COACH

_____

_____

37

Health Partner's Guide 63

SESSION SIX

FRESH AIR

Target time: 30 - 60 Minutes

The Whole Life Health Partner's Guide

 ## BE PREPARED

- [ ] Review the Pre-Session Checklist on page 15 of this guide.
- [ ] Review any information you have on your new friend.
- [ ] Review Session Six completely.
- [ ] Check all electronics to make sure they are charged and working.
- [ ] Pray before you leave to go to the appointment.
- [ ] Video to play: Air
- [ ] **Bring your walking shoes.**

Upon Arrival

Come to the door with a smile. Give them a warm greeting and ask them how they are doing.

 It's time for a walk. Don't forget, this is a wonderful time to get to know them on a personal level and build a friendship. Be open with them and they will be open with you. At this point, they might ask you about your faith. Let the Lord lead you.

 Log Review

Once you are back from your walk, review their weekly log from the previous week on pages **36 and 37. Don't forget to review their meal log. Have them show you that they completed the thankfulness log. This may be private so just check for completion.** Congratulate them if they met their goal(s).

 IF THEY DID NOT MAKE THEIR GOAL(S) SAY THIS:

"I'm sorry you didn't complete your goal(s). Don't be discouraged. You are making progress, and you will get there. Do you think your goal(s) was too big?"

 If yes, ask them if they would like to change the goal(s) to something they know they can do this week.

 If no, ask them if they want to keep the same goal(s) and try it again this week.

 Set the water, activity, nutrition, sleep, and sunlight goal for that week on page 38 and 39.

 Push play on your laptop or DVD player. Only play the **Fresh Air** video.

 Stop the video.
There are no more videos in this session.

Health Partner's Guide 66

SESSION SIX
FRESH AIR

- Review the key points from the video. You should take turns reading them.

- Have them fill out these two sections.

- Have them read the **Four Tips for Success**.

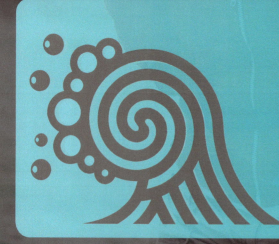

Negative ions tend to concentrate near rivers, waterfalls, and the ocean due to water movement. They also exist in forests, and areas that have just been struck by lightning. These places have up to ten times more negative ions than most homes.[1]

Health Partner's Guide

Negative ions are also referred to as "happy ions" because they contribute to better moods, better energy, and a better sense of wellbeing.[2]

People who spend large amounts of time in places with high negative ion concentration are less likely to be depressed, they have better sleep, and have more energy.[2]

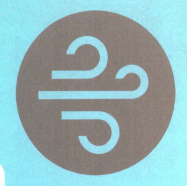

The best air to breath for optimum health is oxygen-rich, negatively charged air.

HOW IS THE AMOUNT OF FRESH AIR YOU ARE GETTING NOW AFFECTING YOUR HEALTH?

HOW WILL BREATHING MORE NEGATIVELY CHARGED AIR AFFECT YOUR CURRENT HEALTH?

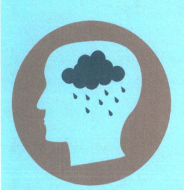

Positive ions have been associated with higher levels of anxiety and depression.[3]

FOUR TIPS TO HELP YOU SUCCEED IN WEEK SIX:

1. Go to a place where there are high concentrations of negative ions, like a forest or the beach. Please, don't go chasing lightning.
2. Step outside for a minute or two every hour for a literal breather. This will help you think clearer and work more efficiently.
3. Sleep with a window opened at night.
4. Grow indoor plants that have large surface areas.

21

Health Partner's Guide **69**

Have them set this week's fresh air goal on **page 40** of the Wellness Planner. Make sure their goal is **S.M.A.R.T.**

 SUGGESTED QUESTIONS FOR SETTING GOALS:

How much fresh air do you get now?

How much fresh air can you add to your daily routine?

How will you add that amount fresh air into your day?

 WRAP IT UP! The session is almost over.

 READ ME: "That is all for today. Be sure and complete all of the logs this week. It is very important for us to see and track all of your progress."

 Confirm the day and time for next week. Give a warm, friendly goodbye. The session is now over.

 Once you leave, complete the Post-Session Checklist on page 16 of this guide.

Health Partner's Guide

What is your fresh air goal for this week?

_____

Daily Fresh Air Log

Example of Daily Fresh Air Log

10 min.	10 min.	15 min.	15 min.	20 min.	25 min.	30 min.

ASK THE COACH

_____

Health Partner's Guide

SESSION SEVEN
TEMPERANCE

Target time: 30 - 60 Minutes

The Whole Life Health Partner's Guide

 ## BE PREPARED

- [ ] Review the Pre-Session Checklist on page 15 of this guide.
- [ ] Review any information you have on your new friend.
- [ ] Review Session Seven completely.
- [ ] Check all electronics to make sure they are charged and working.
- [ ] Pray before you leave to go to the appointment.
- [ ] Video to play: Temperance
- [ ] **Bring your walking shoes.**

UPON ARRIVAL

Come to the door with a smile. Give them a warm greeting and ask them how they are doing.

It's time for a walk. Remember that this is a time to connect with them on a personal level. At this point, they might ask you about your faith. Let the Lord lead you.

Log Review

Once you are back from your walk, review their weekly log from the previous week on **pages 38-40. Don't forget to review their meal log. Have them show you that they completed the thankfulness log. This may be private so just check for completion**. Congratulate them if they met their goal(s).

IF THEY DID NOT MAKE THEIR GOAL(S) SAY THIS:

"I'm sorry you didn't complete your goal(s). Don't be discouraged. You are making progress, and you will get there. Do you think your goal(s) was too big?"

If yes, ask them if they would like to change the goal(s) to something they know they can do this week.

If no, ask them if they want to keep the same goal(s) and try it again this week.

Set the water, activity, nutrition, sleep, sunlight, and fresh air goal for that week on pages 41-42.

Push play on your laptop or DVD player.
Only play the **temperance** video.

Stop the video.
There are no more videos in this session.

Health Partner's Guide 74

- Review the key points from the video. You should take turns reading them.

- Have them fill out these six sections.

- Where are the tips? Being that intemperance can encompass such a broad spectrum, we are leaving it up to you to help them come up with strategies to overcome their obstacles.

"Joy, temperance, and repose slammed the door on the doctor's nose."
—H.W. Longfellow

Health Partner's Guide 76

How are your day-to-day choices affecting your health?
_____
_____

How will being more temperate affect your current health?
_____
_____

What are some habits you know you need to change but cannot seem to get control of?
_____
_____

What positive outcomes can you expect once you gain control over those habits?
_____
_____

How will these new, good habits affect your relationship with others?
_____
_____

How much money, if any, will you save each year by eliminating these bad habits and what would you do with the extra money?
_____
_____

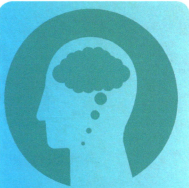

Temperance is a state of mind that gives you balance and control in your life.

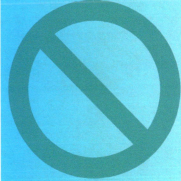

The principle of temperance is this: Eliminate what is bad and moderate what is good.

23

Health Partner's Guide 77

Have them set this week's temperance goal on page 43 of the Wellness Planner. Make sure their goal is **S.M.A.R.T.**

 WRAP IT UP! The session is almost over.

 READ ME: "That is all for today. Be sure and complete all of the logs this week. It is very important for us to see and track all of your progress."

 Confirm the day and time for next week. Give a warm, friendly goodbye. The session is now over.

 Once you leave, complete the Post-Session Checklist on page 16 of this guide.

What is your temperance goal for this week?

_____

_____

Daily Temperance Log

Example of Daily Temperance Log

10 cig	5 cig	2 cig	0 cig	5 AB	4 AB	3 AB

ASK THE COACH _____

_____

Health Partner's Guide

SESSION EIGHT

TRUST IN DIVINE POWER

Target time: 30 - 60 Minutes

The Whole Life Health Partner's Guide

 ## BE PREPARED

- [ ] Review the Pre-Session Checklist on page 15 of this guide.
- [ ] Review any information you have on your new friend.
- [ ] Review Session Eight completely.
- [ ] Check all electronics to make sure they are charged and working.
- [ ] Pray before you leave to go to the appointment.
- [ ] Video to play: Trust in Divine Power
- [ ] **Bring your walking shoes.**

Upon Arrival

Come to the door with a smile. Give them a warm greeting and ask them how they are doing.

It's time for a walk. Remember that this is a time to connect with them on a personal level. At this point, they might ask you about your faith. Let the Lord lead you.

Log Review

Once you are back from your walk, review their weekly log from the previous week on **pages 41-43. Don't forget to review their meal log. Have them show you that they completed the thankfulness log. This may be private so just check for completion.** Congratulate them if they met their goal(s).

IF THEY DID NOT MAKE THEIR GOAL(S) SAY THIS:

"I'm sorry you didn't complete your goal(s). Don't be discouraged. You are making progress, and you will get there. Do you think your goal(s) was too big?"

If yes, ask them if they would like to change the goal(s) to something they know they can do this week.

If no, ask them if they want to keep the same goal(s) and try it again this week.

Set the water, activity, nutrition, sleep, sunlight, fresh air, and temperance goal for that week on pages 44-46.

Push play on your laptop or DVD player. Only play the **Trust in Divine Power** video.

Stop the video.
There are no more videos in this session.

Health Partner's Guide **83**

SESSION EIGHT
TRUST IN DIVINE POWER

 Review the key points from the video. You should take turns reading them.

 Have them fill out these three sections.

 Time to share! If appropriate, this is a perfect time for you to share a short testimony about how prayer has positively impacted your life. If possible, think of something that they can relate to. If they need milk give them milk. If they need meat give them meat.

> Meditation and prayer play important roles in strengthening circuits in our brains. This makes us more socially aware and alert while reducing anxiety, depression, and neurological stress.[1]

Health Partner's Guide 84

Different studies have shown a connection between a lack of religious service attendance and the likelihood of having respiratory disease, infectious diseases, and diabetes. The health risks extend so far as to high blood pressure, depression, suicide, lung cancer, coronary heart disease, chronic obstructive lung disease, and more hospital admissions. You are also more likely to become physically disabled and suffer from a weaker immune system.[2]

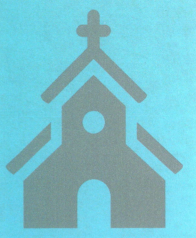

The health benefits of regularly attending religious activities is comparable to not smoking.[2]

LIST SOME THINGS YOU LEARNED ABOUT TRUSTING IN GOD THAT YOU DIDN'T KNOW BEFORE:

HOW DOES/WOULD PRAYING FOR YOURSELF AND OTHERS AFFECT YOUR CURRENT HEALTH?

WHAT POSITIVE OUTCOMES CAN YOU EXPECT IF YOU BEGAN PRAYING TODAY?

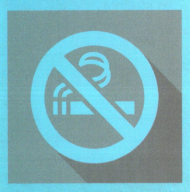

Regular church attendees are more likely to stop smoking, and stay married.[2]

Have them set this week's prayer goal on **page 46** in the Wellness Planner. Make sure their goal is **S.M.A.R.T.** If they already pray regularly, maybe reading the Bible regularly is another goal they could go for.

 WRAP IT UP! The session is almost over.

 READ ME: "That is all for today. Be sure and complete all of the logs this week. It is very important for us to see and track all of your progress. Do you mind if I pray for you right now?"

 IF THEY SAY "YES," SAY THIS:

"Is there anything in particular you would like me to pray about?"

 IF THEY SAY "NO," SAY THIS:

"That's okay. If you change your mind, let me know. I'm here to help you as much as possible in as many ways as possible."

 Confirm the day and time for next week. Give a warm, friendly goodbye. The session is now over.

 Once you leave, complete the Post-Session Checklist on page 16 of this guide.

What is your temperance goal for this week?

_____

_____

Daily Temperance Log

What is your prayer goal for this week?

_____

_____

Daily Prayer Log

Example of Daily Prayer Log

2 min.	2 min.	2 min.	5 min.	5 min.	5 min.	10 min.

Ask the Coach

_____

_____

Health Partner's Guide 87

SESSION NINE
HYGIENE
Target time: 30 - 60 Minutes

The Whole Life Health Partner's Guide

 ## BE PREPARED

- [ ] Review the Pre-Session Checklist on page 15 of this guide.

- [ ] Review any information you have on your new friend.

- [ ] Review Session Nine completely.

- [ ] Check all electronics to make sure they are charged and working.

- [ ] Pray before you leave to go to the appointment.

- [ ] No video today.

- [ ] **Bring your walking shoes.**

Upon Arrival

Come to the door with a smile. Give them a warm greeting and ask them how they are doing.

 It's time for a walk. Remember that this is a time to connect with them on a personal level. Considering last week's session, they might ask you about your faith. Feel free to be open with them. Focus on the positive experiences in your Christian walk and *stay away from doctrines that may be controversial.*

 Log Review

Once you are back from your walk, review their weekly log from the previous week on **pages 44-46. Don't forget to review their meal log. Have them show you that they completed the thankfulness log. This may be private so just check for completion.** Congratulate them if they met their goal(s).

 IF THEY DID NOT MAKE THEIR GOAL(S) SAY THIS:

"I'm sorry you didn't complete your goal(s). Don't be discouraged. You are making progress, and you will get there. Do you think your goal(s) was too big?"

 If yes, ask them if they would like to change the goal(s) to something they know they can do this week.

 If no, ask them if they want to keep the same goal(s) and try it again this week.

 Set the water, activity, nutrition, sleep, sunlight, fresh air, temperance, prayer goal for that week on pages 47-49.

 Read through the material on hygiene on pages 27 and 28 in the Wellness Planner. Taking turns is a great idea!

Personal hygiene plays a crucial role in health and longevity. Keeping your body and your environment clean and tidy will help you in many ways. Here is a list of ways personal hygiene can help your physical, mental, and social health:

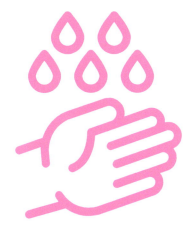

Many diseases and conditions are spread by not washing hands with soap and clean, running water.

Brushing your teeth and flossing daily can save you from pain, embarrassment, and spending thousands of dollars on false teeth in your later years. Not brushing and flossing your teeth daily can lead to gingivitis, gum disease, lung disease, and heart disease.[1]

Bathing daily has a powerful impact on your health. As we go through the day, our skin is constantly shedding and releasing toxins through tiny glands, which if not removed through bathing, can produce a foul odor and breed bacteria. If these bacteria find their way into your mouth, nose, or eyes, you can become ill. Bathing daily will also help you to have good social health, job security, and increase your influence with those around you.

Washing your hands when you touch something that is questionable or after sneezing, coughing, or shaking hands with someone is also good practice. Keeping your nails trimmed and clean eliminates a host of bacteria that can accumulate under them.

Doing laundry, sweeping, mopping, and vacuuming regularly is vital to maintain a good, healthy life. Washing your clothes when soiled will help remove bacteria that can build up from contact with your skin. Washing your bedsheets and pillowcases, bath towels, and kitchen towels on a weekly basis will help fight the spreading of disease and decrease foul odors in your home.

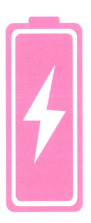

As people clean up, their energy seems to rise.
— Cindy Glovinsky MSW

27

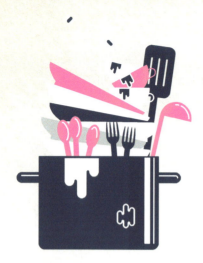

Clutter can actually make it more difficult to focus on a particular task.

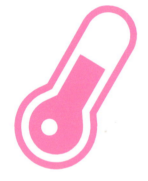

Cooked food that is left in the "danger zone," 40°F–140°F, for more than two hours is considered "unsafe" by the USDA.

Food storage and kitchen cleanliness is well worth mentioning. The Center for Disease Control estimates that each year 48 million people get sick from a food-borne illness, 128,000 are hospitalized, and 3,000 die. Researchers have identified more than 250 foodborne diseases. Cooked food that is left in the "danger zone," 40°F-140°F, for more than two hours is considered "unsafe" by the USDA. Be sure not to let raw or undercooked animal products touch other foods. Designating a specific knife and cutting board and immediately scrubbing it with hot, soapy water is a good practice when handling raw animal products. Cleaning your dishes and wiping the counters and dinner table after each meal will help you keep bacteria under control. It will also help you avoid the stress of seeing a huge pile of dishes at the end of the day.[2]

Julia Cameron said, "When we clear the physical clutter from our lives, we literally make way for inspiration and 'good, orderly direction' to enter." Cluttered surroundings make it difficult to think and make good decisions, they cause anxiety, and make us less productive—Not to mention the dust they accumulate which lessens the air quality.

This may seem like a long list, but not everything mentioned above needs to be done every day. Some things can be done weekly, some monthly, some yearly. It might be a good idea to complete tasks on Thursdays and Fridays. This will allow you to spend quality time on the weekends with friends and family and simply unplug from the hustle and bustle of the work week and just rest.

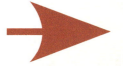

SESSION NINE
HYGIENE

 Have them fill out these four sections.

 Time to help! If there are some projects they need help with, and you are able, let them know you are here to help.

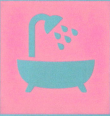 Bathing regularly can reduce stress, inflammation, and muscle pain, while improving your breathing, immune system, and heart health.

Health Partner's Guide 94

HOW ARE YOUR CURRENT HYGIENE HABITS AFFECTING YOUR HEALTH?

_____

_____

_____

HOW WILL KEEPING YOUR BODY AND YOUR ENVIRONMENT CLEAN AND TIDY AFFECT YOUR CURRENT HEALTH?

_____

_____

_____

ARE THERE ANY DEEP CLEANING OR DECLUTTERING PROJECTS YOU WANT TO COMPLETE?

_____

_____

_____

ARE THERE ANY CHANGES YOU WOULD LIKE TO MAKE TO HAVE BETTER HYGIENE?

_____

_____

_____

Have them set this week's hygiene goal on page 49 of the Wellness Planner. Use what they wrote on page 29 to set their goal. Make sure their goal is **S.M.A.R.T. There is no example for this goal on page 49.** This goal can be for personal hygiene, home cleanliness, or even cleaning out the junk drawer that they have been putting off.

 WRAP IT UP! The session is almost over.

 READ ME: "That is all for today. Be sure and complete all of the logs this week. It is very important for us to see and track all of your progress."

 Pray with them if they are open to it.

 Confirm the day and time for next week. Give a warm, friendly goodbye. The session is now over.

 **Once you leave,** complete the Post-Session Checklist on page 16 of this guide.

Health Partner's Guide **96**

What is your temperance goal for this week?

_____

_____

Daily Temperance Log

What is your prayer goal for this week?

_____

_____

Daily Prayer Log

What is your hygiene goal for this week?

_____

_____

Daily Hygiene Log

ASK THE COACH

_____

_____

49

SESSION TEN
MAINTENANCE

Target time: 30 - 60 Minutes

The Whole Life Health Partner's Guide

 ## BE PREPARED

- ☐ Review the Pre-Session Checklist on page 15 of this guide.
- ☐ Review any information you have on your new friend.
- ☐ Review Session Ten completely.
- ☐ Pray before you leave to go to the appointment.
- ☐ No video today.
- ☐ **Bring your walking shoes.**

UPON ARRIVAL

Come to the door with a smile. Give them a warm greeting and ask them how they are doing.

It's time for a walk. Remember that this is a time to connect with them on a personal level. If they are still not open to talk about spiritual topics, don't be pushy. If they are open, be sure not to over water the seeds.

Log Review

Once you are back from your walk, review their weekly log from the previous week on **pages 47-49. Don't forget to review their meal log. Have them show you that they completed the thankfulness log. This may be private so just check for completion.** Congratulate them if they met their goal(s).

IF THEY DID NOT MAKE THEIR GOAL(S) SAY THIS:

"I'm sorry you didn't complete your goal(s). Don't be discouraged. You are making progress, and you will get there. Do you think your goal(s) was too big?"

If yes, ask them if they would like to change the goal(s) to something they know they can do this week.

If no, ask them if they want to keep the same goal(s) and try it again this week.

Have them set goals for this week on pages 50-52.

Health Partner's Guide

WRAP IT UP! The session is almost over.

 READ ME: "That is all for today."

 Pray with them if they are open to it.

 Confirm the day and time for next week. Give a warm, friendly goodbye. The session is now over.

 Once you leave, complete the Post-Session Checklist on page 16 of this guide.

SESSION ELEVEN
MAINTENANCE

Target time: 30 - 60 Minutes

The Whole Life Health Partner's Guide

 ## BE PREPARED

- [ ] Review the Pre-Session Checklist on page 15 of this guide.
- [ ] Review any information you have on your new friend.
- [ ] Review Session Eleven completely.
- [ ] Pray before you leave to go to the appointment.
- [ ] No video today.
- [ ] **Bring your walking shoes.**

Upon Arrival

Come to the door with a smile. Give them a warm greeting and ask them how they are doing.

It's time for a walk. Remember that this is a time to connect with them on a personal level. If they are still not open to talk about spiritual topics, don't be pushy. If they are open, be sure not to over water the seeds.

Log Review

Once you are back from your walk, review their weekly log from the previous week on **pages 50-52. Don't forget to review their meal log. Have them show you that they completed the thankfulness log. This may be private so just check for completion.** Congratulate them if they met their goal(s).

IF THEY DID NOT MAKE THEIR GOAL(S) SAY THIS:

"I'm sorry you didn't complete your goal(s). Don't be discouraged. You are making progress, and you will get there. Do you think your goal(s) was too big?"

If yes, ask them if they would like to change the goal(s) to something they know they can do this week.

If no, ask them if they want to keep the same goal(s) and try it again this week.

Have them set goals for this week on pages 53-55.

Health Partner's Guide 104

WRAP IT UP! The session is almost over.

 READ ME: "That is all for today."

 Pray with them if they are open to it.

 Confirm the day and time for next week. Give a warm, friendly goodbye. The session is now over.

 Once you leave, complete the Post-Session Checklist on page 16 of this guide.

SESSION TWELVE
MAINTENANCE
Target time: 30 - 60 Minutes

The Whole Life Health Partner's Guide

 ## BE PREPARED

- ☐ Review the Pre-Session Checklist on page 15 of this guide.

- ☐ Review any information you have on your new friend.

- ☐ Review Session Twelve completely.

- ☐ Pray before you leave to go to the appointment.

- ☐ No video today.

- ☐ **Bring your walking shoes.**

- ☐ **Bring the Certificate of Completion.**

Upon Arrival

Come to the door with a smile. Give them a warm greeting and ask them how they are doing.

It's time for a walk. Remember that this is a time to connect with them on a personal level. If they are still not open to talk about spiritual topics, don't be pushy. If they are open, be sure not to over water the seeds.

Log Review

Once you are back from your walk, review their weekly log from the previous week on **pages 53-55. Don't forget to review their meal log. Have them show you that they completed the thankfulness log. This may be private so just check for completion.** Congratulate them if they met their goal(s).

IF THEY DID NOT MAKE THEIR GOAL(S) SAY THIS:

"I'm sorry you didn't complete your goal(s). Don't be discouraged. You are making progress, and you will get there. Do you think your goal(s) was too big?"

If yes, ask them if they would like to change the goal(s) to something they know they can do this week.

If no, ask them if they want to keep the same goal(s) and try it again this week.

Have them set goals for this week on pages 56-58.

WRAP IT UP! The session is almost over.

 READ ME: "I have really enjoyed our time together. Since you have completed the twelfth session, I am honored to present to you The Whole Life's Certificate of Completion for twelve weeks of coaching [give them the certificate]. How has your journey to the whole life been?

As I mentioned to you in the beginning, at the end of the twelfth session, we would reassess and see if you want to continue. Do you think that is something that would benefit you?"

 IF "YES", SAY THIS: "Great! I can order you a new planner this week. Do you want to pay me now or when I come back? Also, just use the extra logs until the new planner comes in.

Also, there is another activity that is part of program that we like to offer people and that is The Whole Life Bible Study Book. Is that something you might be interested in also?"

 IF "NO", SAY THIS: "That is okay. This sadly means that this is our last session. However, if you ever want to do this again feel free to call me and we could start again. Also, there is another activity that is a sequel of this program. It is The Whole Life Bible Study Book. Is that something you might be interested in?" Pray with them if they are open to it.

 IF "YES", SAY THIS: "Great! Will the same day and time work? If you want, we can walk a little before each study."

Health Partner's Guide

IF "NO", SAY THIS: "That's okay too. If you change your mind don't be afraid to ask. I want to thank you for allowing me to be part of your life for the past 12 weeks. I hope this isn't the end of our friendship."

 Give a warm, friendly goodbye. The session is now over.

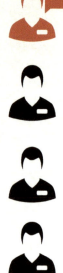 **Once you leave,** complete the Post-Session Checklist on page 16 of this guide.

 Order the materials needed.

Health Partner's Guide 110

NOTES

NOTES

Work Cited

Water

[1] *American Journal of Epidemiology*, Volume 155, Issue 9, 1 May 2002, Pages 827–833,

[2] Ferraro PM, Taylor EN, Gambaro G, Curhan GC. Dietary and lifestyle risk factors associated with incident kidney stones in men and women. J Urol. 2017;198(4):858-863. PMID: 28365271

[3] Math MV, Rampal PM, Faure XR, Delmont JP. Gallbladder emptying after drinking water and its possible role in prevention of gallstone formation. Singapore Med J (in press).

[4] National Digestive Diseases Information Clearinghouse (NDDIC): "Constipation," and "What I Need to Know About Constipation."

[5] National Institute of Diabetes and Digestive and Kidney Diseases (NIDDK) https://www.niddk.nih.gov/health-information/urologic-diseases/bladder-infection-uti-in-adults/treatment

[6] Reporter, VANDERBILT UNIVERSITY MEDICAL CENTER'S WEEKLY NEWSPAPER, "Plain water has surprising impact on blood pressure", BY: LEIGH MACMILLAN 7/08/2010

[7] International Glaucoma Association,"Lifestyle - Will it help or hinder your glaucoma?"
https://www.glaucoma-association.com/about-glaucoma/living-with-glaucoma/lifestyle/, This article is based on a talk given at the IGA Glaucoma Support Group meeting at Addenbrookes Hospital, Cambridge, in October 2015.

[8] Texas Heart Institute, Venous blood clots (including DVT), https://www.texasheart.org/heart-health/heart-information-center/topics/venous-blood-clots/

Work Cited

Activity

[1] Steven C. Moore, Alpa V. Patel, Charles E. Matthews, Amy Berrington de Gonzalez, Yikyung Park, Hormuzd A. Katki, Martha S. Linet, Elisabete Weiderpass, Kala Visvanathan, Kathy J. Helzlsouer, Michael Thun, Susan M. Gapstur, Patricia Hartge, I-Min Lee *Leisure Time Physical Activity of Moderate to Vigorous Intensity and Mortality: A Large Pooled Cohort Analysis, Published* November 6, 2012. https://doi.org/10.1371/journal.pmed.1001335

[2] Venturelli M, Schena F, Richardson RS. The role of exercise capacity in the health and longevity of centenarians. *Maturitas.* 2012;73(2):115-20.

[3] U.S. Department of Health and Human Services. Physical Activity Guidelines for Americans, 2nd edition. Washington, DC: U.S. Department of Health and Human Services; 2018.

[4] Mandsager K, Harb S, Cremer P, Phelan D, Nissen SE, Jaber W. Association of Cardiorespiratory Fitness With Long-term Mortality Among Adults Undergoing Exercise Treadmill Testing. *JAMA Netw Open.*2018;1(6):e183605. doi:10.1001/jamanetworkopen.2018.3605

[5] Hirsch CH, Diehr P, Newman AB, et al. Physical activity and years of healthy life in older adults: results from the cardiovascular health study. *J Aging Phys Act.* 2010;18(3):313-34.

[6] Dieli-Conwright CM, Lee K, Kiwata JL. Reducing the Risk of Breast Cancer Recurrence: an Evaluation of the Effects and Mechanisms of Diet and Exercise. *Curr Breast Cancer Rep.* 2016;8(3):139-150.

Nutrition

[1] 8 Laws of Health DVD, Chapter 4, Nutrition

Work Cited

Sleep

[1] National Sleep Foundation https://www.sleep.org/articles/how-long-you-sleep-impacts-weight/ The surprising connection between hours clocked sleeping and what the scale says

[2] News release, American Academy of Sleep Medicine.
24th annual meeting of the Associated Professional Sleep Societies LLC, San Antonio, June 6-9, 2010. *Morbidity and Mortality Weekly Report*; Oct. 30, 2009; vol 58(42): pp 1175-1179.

[3] Bivens, Randy MD, 8 Laws of Health DVD, Chapter 5, Rest

[4] Brain basics: Understanding sleep. (2019). ninds.nih.gov/disorders/brain_basics/understanding_sleep.htm

[5] β-Amyloid accumulation in the human brain after one night of sleep deprivation. Shokri-Kojori E, Wang GJ, Wiers CE, Demiral SB, Guo M, Kim SW, Lindgren E, Ramirez V, Zehra A, Freeman C, Miller G, Manza P, Srivastava T, De Santi S, Tomasi D, Benveniste H, Volkow ND. Proc Natl Acad Sci USA. 2018 Apr 9. pii: 201721694. doi: 10.1073/pnas.1721694115. [Epub ahead of print] PMID: 29632177.

[6] Diwakar Balachandran, MD, director, Sleep Center, University of Texas M.D. Anderson Cancer Center, Houston.
John Park, MD, pulmonologist, Mayo Clinic, Rochester, Minn.
Susan Zafarlotfi, PhD, clinical director, Institute for Sleep and Wake Disorders, Hackensack University Medical Center, N.J.
Morbidity and Mortality Weekly Report, Oct. 30, 2009; vol 58: pp 1171-1198.

[7] Hublin C, Partinen M, Koskenvuo M, Kaprio J. Sleep and mortality: a population-based 22-year follow-up study. Sleep. 2007;30(10):1245–1253.

[8] Gooley JJ, Chamberlain K, Smith KA, et al. Exposure to room light before bedtime suppresses melatonin onset and shortens melatonin duration in humans. *J Clin Endocrinol Metab.* 2010;96(3):E463–E472. doi:10.1210/jc.2010-2098

WORK CITED

[9] Pagel JF, Parnes BL. Medications for the Treatment of Sleep Disorders: An Overview. *Prim Care Companion J Clin Psychiatry*. 2001;3(3):118–125.

SUNSHINE

[1] Holick MF. Resurrection of vitamin D deficiency and rickets. *J Clin Invest*. 2006;116(8):2062–2072. doi:10.1172/JCI29449

[2] Sunyecz JA. The use of calcium and vitamin D in the management of osteoporosis. *Ther Clin Risk Manag*. 2008;4(4):827–836.

[3] *The American Journal of Clinical Nutrition*, Volume 79, Issue 3, March 2004, Pages 362–371, https://doi.org/10.1093/ajcn/79.3.362
Published: 01 March 2004

[4] Wacker M, Holick MF. Sunlight and Vitamin D: A global perspective for health. Dermatoendocrinol. 2013;5(1):51–108. doi:10.4161/derm.24494

[5] Meesters Y, Gordijn MC. Seasonal affective disorder, winter type: current insights and treatment options. *Psychol Res Behav Manag*. 2016;9:317–327. Published 2016 Nov 30. doi:10.2147/PRBM.S114906

FRESH AIR

[1] Jiang SY, Ma A, Ramachandran S. Negative Air Ions and Their Effects on Human Health and Air Quality Improvement. *Int J Mol Sci*. 2018;19(10):2966. Published 2018 Sep 28. doi:10.3390/ijms19102966

[2] Perez V, Alexander DD, Bailey WH. Air ions and mood outcomes: a review and meta-analysis. *BMC Psychiatry*. 2013;13:29. Published 2013 Jan 15. doi:10.1186/1471-244X-13-29

[3] J Clin Psychiatry. Giannini AJ, Jones BT, Loiselle RH. 1986 Mar;47(3):141-3. *Reversibility of serotonin irritation syndrome with atmospheric anions*. https://www.ncbi.nlm.nih.gov/pubmed/3949723

Work Cited

Trust in Divine Power

[1] Newberg, Andrew MD, Waldman, Mark R. (2009) *How God Changes Your Brain*, New York, Ballentine Books

[2] Koenig HG. Religion, spirituality, and health: the research and clinical implications. *ISRN Psychiatry*. 2012;2012:278730. Published 2012 Dec 16. doi:10.5402/2012/278730

Hygiene

[1] Makkar H, Reynolds MA, Wadhawan A, Dagdag A, Merchant AT, Postolache TT. Periodontal, metabolic, and cardiovascular disease: Exploring the role of inflammation and mental health. Pteridines. 2018;29(1):124–163. doi:10.1515/pteridines-2018-0013

[2] https://www.cdc.gov/foodsafety/communication/food-safety-in-the-kitchen.html

CPSIA information can be obtained
at www.ICGtesting.com
Printed in the USA
LVHW072304271221
707299LV00004B/69